resilient cadence

A POETRY ANTHOLOGY

MY JOURNEY IN MEDICINE

Megan Y. Kamath, MD

First edition 2026

ISBN (hardcover): 979-8-9961602-0-4
ISBN (paperback): 979-8-9961602-1-1
ISBN (ebook): 979-8-9961602-2-8

ACKNOWLEDGEMENTS

I am deeply grateful to everyone who stood beside me through both the quiet hours of doubt and the bright moments of discovery. To my family and friends—your faith in my words gave them wings. To my mentors and fellow writers—thank you for teaching me that poetry is not only written, but lived.

DEDICATION

For my parents—who taught me the meaning of love, patience, and the quiet power of dreams

For my husband—thank you for the laughter, the encouragement, and for always cheering me on

For my children—may you always chase wonder and find your own voices in the world

For my brother—thank you for reminding me that family is both our roots and our wings

contents

Author's Note: This poem was written by the author at age 8 and originally published in her 3rd grade poetry book. The author wanted to be a physician since the age of 5.

I Am

I am an adventurous girl who wants to be a doctor
I wonder if I will ever become a doctor
I hear patients crying in pain
I see all the people who are sick and want to get better
I want to have a cure for every sickness
I am an adventurous girl who wants to be a doctor

I feel sad when a person dies
I touch the hand of someone who is ill
I worry that I might not become a doctor
I cry when I get pricked by a needle
I am an adventurous girl who wants to be a doctor

I understand that people always get sick
I try to make people feel better
I hope that my dream will come true
I know I will be a good doctor
I am an adventurous girl who wants to be a doctor

The System Works for the System

It's strange, isn't it?
How a place built for healing
can feel so hollow inside.
The lights never dim,
while the people beneath them do.

The system works, but for whom?
It churns, it counts, it files.
It praises efficiency.
But it doesn't groan as our bones do
under the weight
of another patient slipping through the cracks
because the margins didn't balance.
There's a quiet misalignment
between what heals and what's rewarded,
between the oath we took
and the metrics we must meet.

We are the problem
when we bend beneath the strain,
as if compassion were weakness,
as if exhaustion were choice.

The system sees us as expendable—
replaceable parts in a grinding machine
that measures output, not grace.
We were trained to listen for heartbeats,
now we listen to billing codes.
We wanted to stop the bleeding,
now we stop the clock.
We used to speak the language of healing—
now it's policy and compliance.

And yet, somewhere within the noise,
a faint pulse reminds us
why we began.
Something still whispers,
asking us who we are
when the caring costs too much.
How do we turn this tide
that drags us from prevention to repair,
from presence to paperwork?
How do we fight headwinds
that call profit progress
at the expense of people and
relationships and things that matter?

The system works for the system.
But I still want to believe
there's another way—
a quieter medicine,
one that remembers the faces
and the promise beyond the oath.
Until then, I keep showing up.
Not because the system works,
but because somewhere within its wreckage,
a few of us still do—
waiting for dawn to break
through the hospital glass.

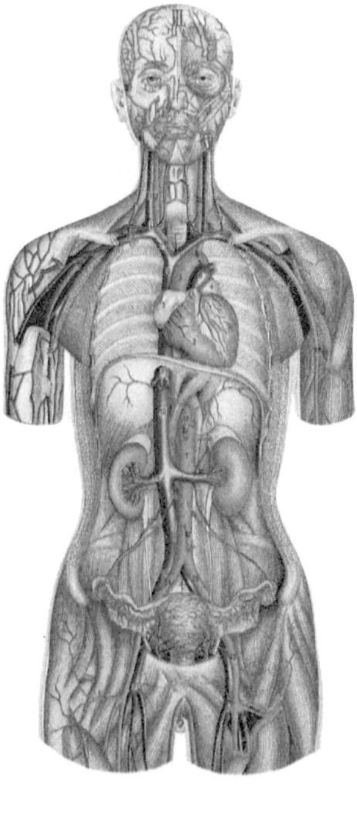

The Graveyard in the Mind

Each doctor carries a graveyard in their head,
with tombstones heavy, unmarked, and unseen.
Names fade like breath on a winter window,
but the silence that follows still remains.
These are not tombs of failure alone.
They are mausoleums full of moments—
hands once held, lungs once
steadied by whispered hope.
Routines conceal the ache:
charts filled, prescriptions signed,
a practiced smile smooths the edges
of the ghosts that linger in the margins.
At night, in the half-light between duty and dream,
they walk the narrow paths of memory,
where angels keep quiet company—
some carrying souls away,
some steadying trembling hands.
For healing means walking beside angels,
one foot in the world of the living,
one brushing the wings of the departed.
And though their hearts are heavy gardens,
they still rise each dawn
to tend what life remains.

Happy Birthing Day

We arrived in the same breath, you and I—
one cry echoing twice through the morning sky.
You, soft and new in the circle of light,
me, remade in your gaze, learning how to be right.
You were the bloom, I the soil turned anew,
roots entwined, growing wild as love tends to do.
I taught you the world; you taught me my heart,
each sunrise reminding how shared beginnings start.
Through laughter and sleepless, wonder-filled nights,
we traded our lessons, our wrongs and our rights.
Two souls born together, not just one hour but all—
each year we remember that sacred first call.
Happy birthing day, my mirrored small flame,
you gave me a title, and I gave you your name.
We are tethered by more than the pull of the years—
made twice in one moment, in laughter and tears.

Introspective Spaces

I had to dig down deep to find
the creativity that awaited to emerge.
Had to go on an artist's date with myself,
to learn a new skill,
to remember what it feels like
to create without a map.
When we are younger,
we step into the unknown with ease—
curious, open, unafraid.
Now I move with more trepidation,
shaped by years of carving
the same path, steering away from change.
To find that restless creative spark
took a gentle length of unlearning.
But now that I've found it,
I cannot leave it behind again.

Practice

Sometimes practice makes us sound uncertain,
As if ten thousand hours still aren't enough.
What defines mastery? A test?
Or a moment of true connection?

Sometimes practice feels like losing ourselves,
We—keepers of sacred trust,
Bound by oaths to care—
Forget our own agency.

Yet practice, when cultivated with love,
Becomes the soil of well-being,
The rhythm that sustains us.

In the end,
We must learn not only to serve,
But to thrive.

Always Remember

There is a person behind every patient.
A mom, a dad, a brother, a sister,
someone's best friend,
the caregiver who never rests,
the maker of the world's best gumbo.
Someone fighting insurance for a sliver of hope,
someone balancing heartbreak and bills,
someone with a hidden gift
for painting, singing, building, healing.
Someone who feeds others
yet forgets to feed themselves.
Someone who needs your care
not just for their body, but their spirit.
Never forget:
this work is relational,
this practice is human.

Acceptable

How is it okay
for you to call me by my first name
in front of everyone,
while I must call you Doctor—
or risk a storm that splits the sky?
How is it okay
for you to phone me,
tell me to cut short the healing,
when you've never bothered
to stitch yourself back together?
How is it okay
for you to claim what I built alone,
your name glinting on work
you had no hand in shaping?
How is it okay
to act like you lead
when your power is only gravity—
pulling others down
to keep your crown steady?

Empowerment

Don't fear the name—
It's time to claim it.
You hold the power.
It's time to own it.
Believe in your flame.
Worth more than the moment,
You rise beyond circumstance.
Thought shapes feeling,
Feeling shapes action.
Pause or move,
Hide or ignite.
Steady state, no—
Choose motion.
Let's go.

All You Have Ever Wanted

For years, this was all you wanted.
Laser-focused, eyes on the end game.
Finally, the summit came near
and you reached the pinnacle—
the grit and toil done—
And now, you wonder what's left to come.
The neural pathways short circuit and flicker—
they have not known anything else
that you could have possibly thought to want.

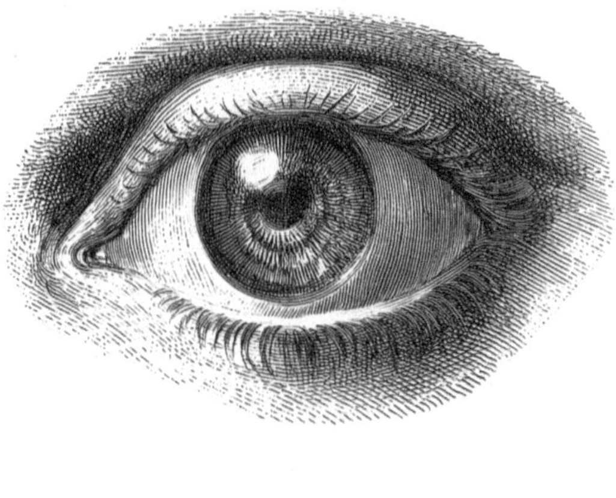

Goodnight Moon

Goodnight, Moon,
with your snaggle-tooth smile.
Will the tooth fairy fly with us awhile?
There, a sprinkle of magic shimmers
on the frosted clouds above,
guiding us softly to dreamland
under a blanket woven with stars and love.
The sweetest dream I'll ever see
is knowing how special you are to me.

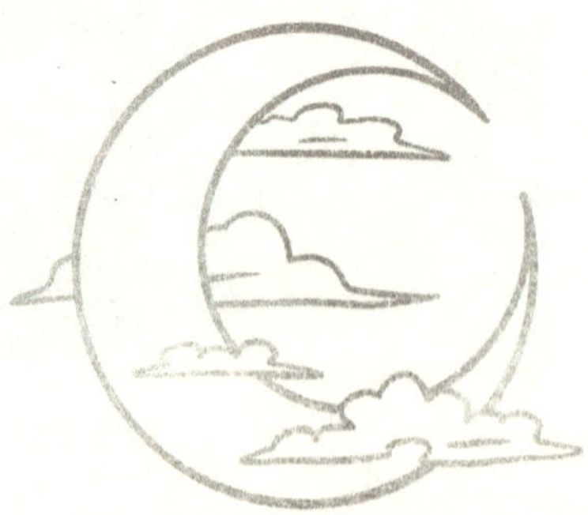

Las Frutas

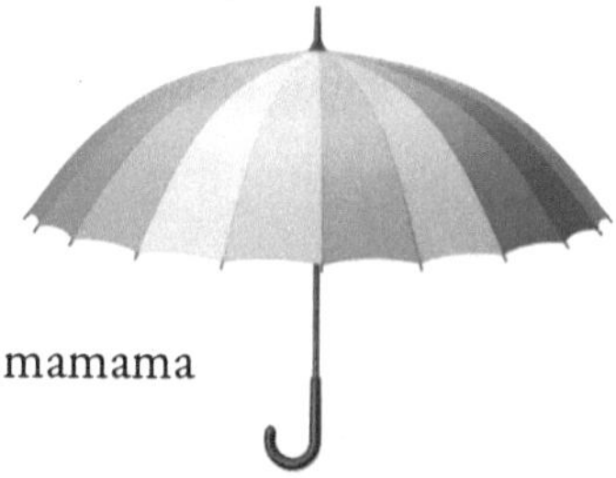

Rainbow umbrella
Green mango
Puckering lips
Refreshing aam panna made by mamama

White young coco
        thud thud
drop from the tall trees in the village.
        The air smells of earth and summer rain.

Yellow nanches and their juicy sunshine
        drip sweet nectar on my fingers.
Orange cantaloupe
        smothered in Tajin and Chamoy
The yin and yang—
Sour, sweet,
Hot, spicy, citrus—
        what memory tastes like.

Love

There is love
And then there is what we share—
a feeling too ancient for the dictionary.
Not *agape*,
not kinship,
no word can describe it.

A fluttering minnow in my stomach,
a connection of cells transforms day by day—
it is an infinite love
woven from starlight,
that began smaller than a grain of sand
and has become the softest,
most precious thing in the world.

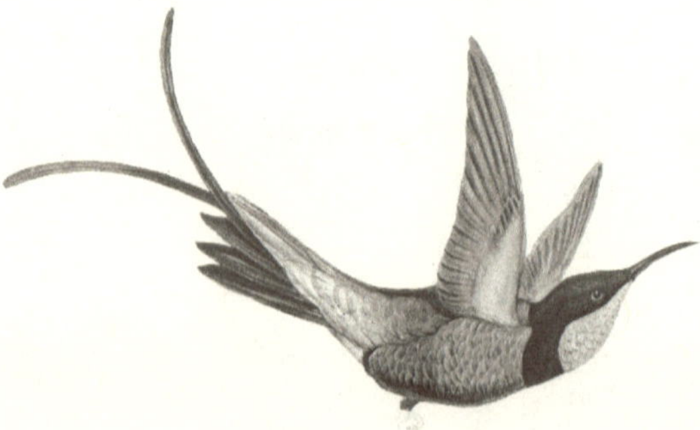

Normal?

Where else is it normal
to not eat or drink,
to not rest
all in the name of care?
Since when was neglecting your body
applauded in the name of service?
Since when did self-destruction
earn a gold medal?
Where in our training were we taught
to forget ourselves so completely?
This system is broken.
We clock in, bloodshot and hungry, for our shifts,
And still, we are told to smile.

Stuck

Thick as honey,
I am suspended in ice—
where is the flow?
Not even a drop,
just the ache of drought.
Can the code be broken,
the spell undone,
to find the magic within?

Feeling

Reach inside and maybe you'll find
the depths of my soul—
restless, still yearning,
tempered by all I've lived.
Burned once by a fire that spread
too fast on the matchstick to hold,
I stand here, waiting,
as the ocean's breath licks at my door.
Come back out—
the tide calls us home.

Guardian

Beneath the great oak—
Its crown full and green,
A guardian of quiet life—
Spring returns again,
A soft whisper of renewal.
A trembling sapling
Faces the wind alone.

I wish you could hear me say,
The world will cradle you;
you'll be okay.
Young maple, learning still,
Your roots now seek the earth.
Reaching, twisting, testing strength—
Not yet tame, but taking form.

Magnolia in bloom,
You've watched the seasons turn.
Night jasmine lingers at your feet,
While a shy orange ripens nearby—
The air is sweet with memory.

And you, steadfast eucalyptus,
With silver skin and whispered scent,
Keeper of countless secrets—
What sights have you gathered,
What worlds await your gaze?

Oh, beautiful being,
Giant, gentle tree—
How lucky we are
To stand beneath your mystery.

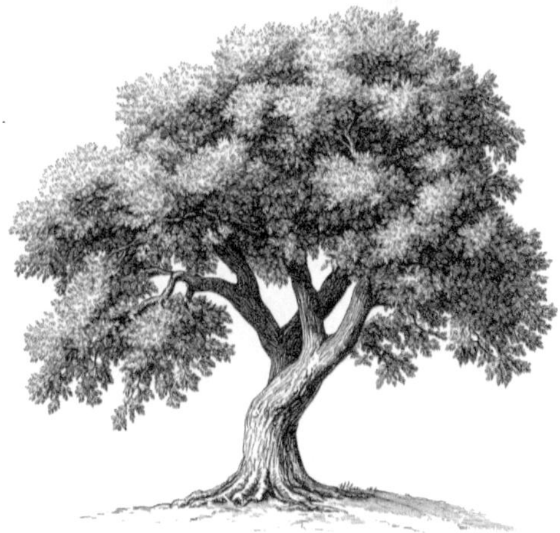

Surrender

Give in to your magical thinking,
And build those castles in the sky.
Climb the beanstalk,
reach for wonders passing by.
Keep the faith and the starlight in view,
For all that is noble and true—
But sometimes, breathe in, then surrender,
And let the universe move you.

Inspire

Some say it's inspiring—
we're proud of you.
It feels like a journey
of a million quiet steps,
meandering, swaying
this way and that.
A gut check.
One foot forward,
then the next.
Reorient, reset,
breathe again.
I'm sorry to read this—
I hoped it would work out.
Still, it's been a real pleasure,
this dance between hope and doubt.
Somewhere beneath it all,
the subconscious stirs—
alive, awake, listening.

In Too Deep

Too far out,
Yet halfway in.
Not far enough,
Yet not fully within.
Running farther,
Then coming near.
The pull remains,
Both bright and clear.

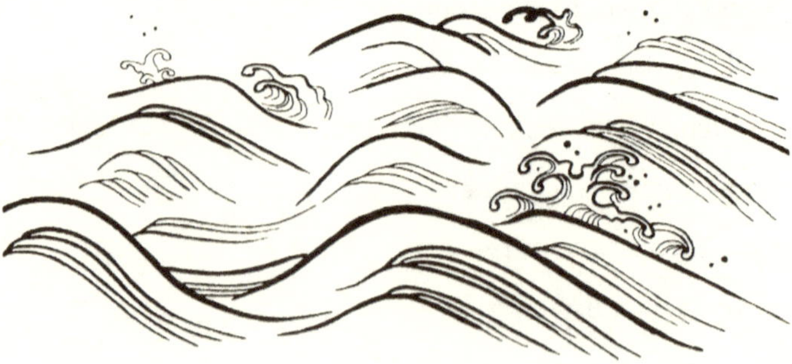

I Miss You

I miss the way you were
But love the way you are.
I wish time would freeze
But love the way you grow:
First, you crawl, then walk—
Soon you'll fly away!
But I will rest assured
That I have taught you
all I know.

Our existence
Alone and together is finite
But to me you are infinite—
We are but children of the cosmos
With divine light shining within.
The love we share between us
Will never be broken.

Fire Horse

A powerful force of nature,
One that is bold and confident,
One that whinnies loudly
With a "I know what I am doing."
A glitter bomb of magic,
Pulsing with youthful glow—
Tenacious spirit unbridled,
Tosses its rainbow mane.
A storm wrapped in sunlight,
Bold and certain of its stride,
Daring the world with a knowing grin.

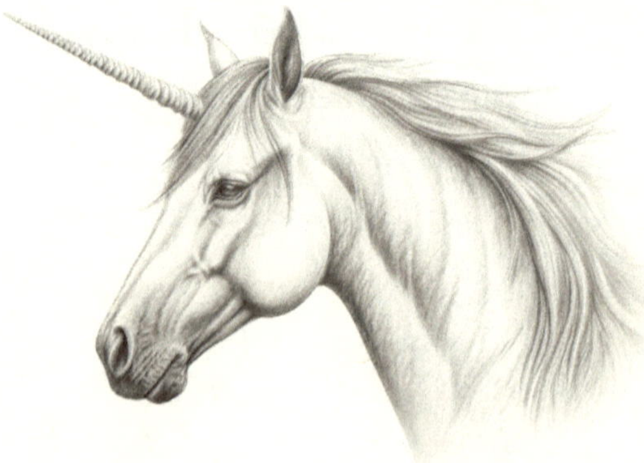

Been There Too

Not the exact same place,
y'know, but I've walked in those shoes.
I've seen the wider view—
the five-year plans,
the ten-year ones,
the lifetime ones.
They've been broken,
bent, rewritten, translated
through love and loss.
Sometimes only experience can sow
the seeds of what's to come—
And guide us toward the harvest
that only time will reveal.

Behind Me

Behind me expands an invisible network,
upon which I've stood to reach this point.
Behind me, a spider's web of collaborations,
Interwoven through six degrees—
Or more—of separation.
In front of me rises a mountain to climb.
Yet I know I can do it,
Because they are with me in spirit,
Speaking softly in my mind,
Echoing through my dreams.
Inside me lives a deep-seated desire
To find meaning and purpose
In healing and in health.
The tree of life sprouts perennially,
Rooted in gratitude,
Renewed in promise.

To Care

What does it truly mean?
To hold another's hand as if it were your own,
To believe in them as fiercely as sunlight fights the dark,
To guide them gently when their path grows dim,
To lift them higher, so they might someday stand on their own?
To know the world is often cruel,
And still choose kindness, again and again?
What does it mean, to truly care?

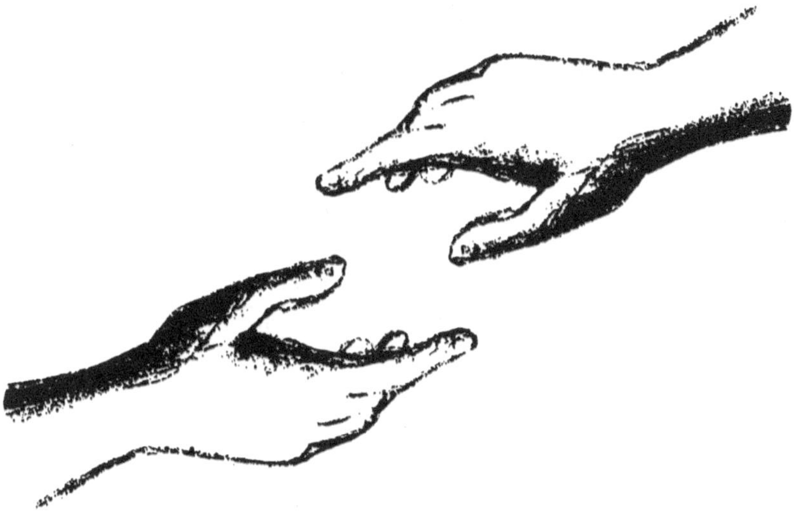

Still

In the stillness I meet myself again—
An unfinished story; a seed still opening.
Growth hums beneath the surface,
a quiet pulse reminding me to keep
reaching and deepening my roots.
A guiding light moves beside me—
encouraging a sacred unfolding of my soul.
Peace does not mean still water—
it means knowing how to flow with the current.
Here, where breath meets trust,
I find belonging in my own unfolding.
I am endlessly whole.

Lift As We Rise

What was once a promise
is now a hollow echo.
The intention was pure,
and for a moment it shone—
until the raging waters came,
a flood, a divine collision
only the universe could design.
In the chaos,
you turned cold,
dismantling me piece by piece—
a shadow that devours.
All that was mine was
erased by your hunger.

What Once Was

What once was
Will never be the same again.
Nothing lasts forever—
Change, the only constant.
An invisible thread,
Binding birth to rebirth,
Tugs at a quiet yearning.
A constellation still forming,
Waiting somewhere between
endings and beginnings.

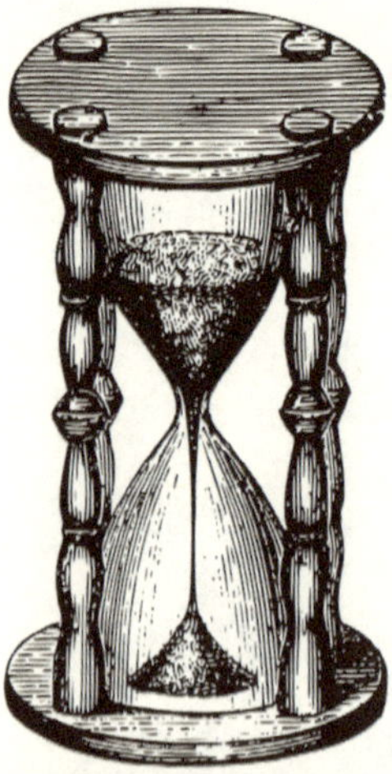

Wise Old Man

Wise old man,
Listening, steady and kind,
Urges me to write—
To find the faint strains of hope
Beneath the weight of anger,
To see the dawn of a new world
Where Rome's ashes still glow.

To doctor is to teach,
To guide, to heal,
A simple creed:
The brightest light still lies ahead.
I await the day
When the journey circles home—
Perhaps once,
I've been there before.

Depth

Your venom carves canyons
deeper than nightmares dared dreamt.
Did Mother ever whisper "manners"?
Clearly not—
you've plummeted past redemption.
Karma's blade swings back,
swift and unyielding,
to carve out your reckoning.

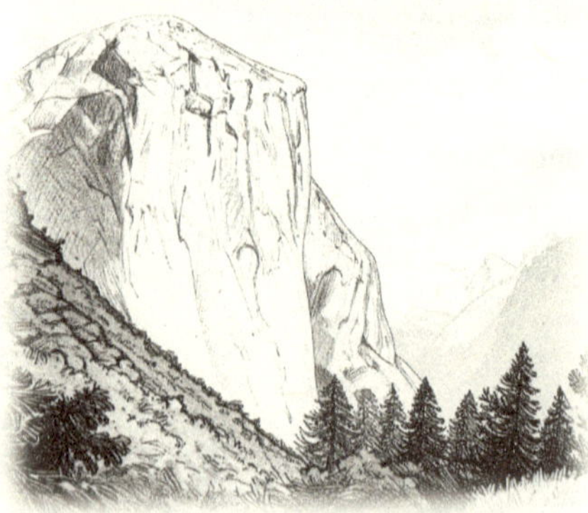

Enjoying the Season

The season of singleness,
of soft love and steady friendship,
of growing quietly into myself.
Of learning what stays,
and what needs to go.
Of bright mornings and longer nights,
of laughter captured in old songs,
of coffee shared with new faces
and comfort with the old.
Of a little sadness too—
the kind that teaches me
how full life can feel
even when it is incomplete.

Missing

A piece is gone—
lost, not found,
and I'm still blind
to where it fell.

Too many sides
to turn over,
too many cracks
to call whole again.
The die was cast
before I even knew
the game had begun.

Time—
healer and executioner—
smears my days
like fingerpaint
on a cracked wall.

A piece is gone—
lost, not found,
and I'm still blind
to where it fell.

Prayer

For guidance,
for peace,
for what is meant to be,
for what will come in time.
In thinking,
in waiting,
in dancing,
in laughter's quiet echo.
For love,
for calm,
for gentle reassurance,
for the stillness of the night
that reminds me—
I am held, even here.

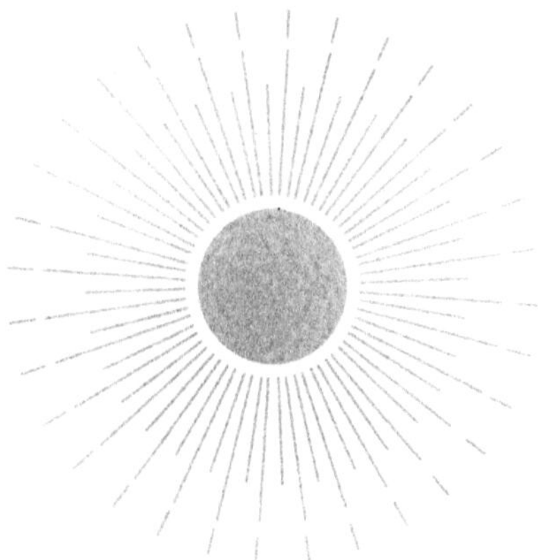

The Time is Right

It's time to make a change.
It feels right—finally—
like releasing a breath
I've been holding too long.

I'll follow my heart for once,
and let the what ifs wait their turn.

It's going to be okay,
one way or another.

If I need to change again,
that's alright too—
we all find our footing,
one step at a time.

Choosing Me

Is this the right thing to do?
Do I just want to end the waiting?
To avoid the unknown in the face
Of what I already know?
Where is the passion—the spark,
the pulse that feels like home?
Will it ever come,
or is "okay" all I can trust?
I cry, unsure why.
Fear hums beneath my ribs—
fear of stillness,
fear of no plan,
fear that nothing guarantees joy.
I once dreamed of passion,
of arrival, of completion.
Realizing it might not come
feels like ballet on broken glass—
grace filled with trembling.
Should I leap or linger?
Move on, or hold my ground
and hope the winds will shift?

I am not unhappy,
but far from ecstatic.
Maybe it's not failure I fear
but the thought
that I could have been more.
The "what ifs" return like ghosts,
whispering through sleepless nights:
Is it time to let go?
Is this my sign?
I just don't know—
and that unknowing
is what shakes me most.

Patience

Through years that burned the tongue,
I learned patience in long fields of yearning.
Seeing both shadows and light—
the bitter served its purpose well.
It carved the vessel, taught me depth,
a quiet craft of knowing who I am.
I've learned to listen past the noise,
to trust the quiet more than the fear.
Growth was patient, never loud,
and stillness carried me here.
Now I stand clear-eyed, unafraid,
steady in what I know.
It's time to cut the bitter,
to eat the sweet.
I know what I am doing,
and the time is right.

Thanks

I called for help,
Not out of weakness,
But with the hope
That someone might understand.
Your disbelief met me
Like a slamming door—
An immediate reminder
That all hearts cannot enter it.
I carried the weight
Of being unwelcome,
Mistaking your silence
For something I'd done wrong.
You said I was resented
For choosing healing.
But healing doesn't ask for permission.
Now I see more clearly—
you taught me by example
everything I no longer wish to be.

Stable

There is relief in restored order—
yet is the absence of motion
the apex of care?
Stasis is not peace,
but merely suspension—
a body anesthetized against its own becoming.
In medicine, stability buys time.
In thought, it spends it.
The mind, too, can flatline
in the name of equilibrium.
Once, change was the measure of vitality;
now stillness is a virtue,
and questioning is treated like infection.
"Stable"—such a clean word
for something so close to decay.

Constellations

A twinkling trail,
like breadcrumbs,
guides the path ahead.
The North Star
frames a vision
of what's to come,
anchoring me
to changing seasons,
the turning pages,
the steady march of time.
Within these patterns,
a shape emerges,
connecting us
to the universe.

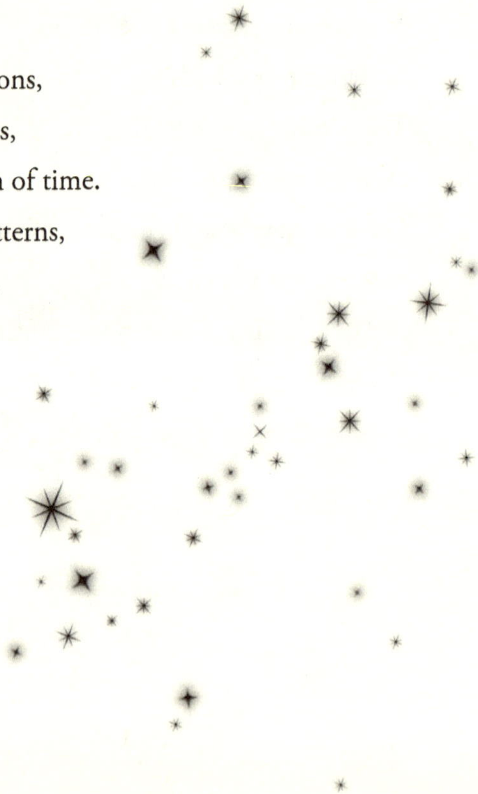

Multiplied

If you have never held
two lives at once—
one in your arms,
one with your hands—
you may not understand
how the weight is the same.
How both can tremble.
How both can trust you completely.

I know the rhythm of a lullaby
and the rhythm of ventricular tachycardia.
I know how to rock
and how to resuscitate.
If you have never stood
in a doorway in the early morning hours
trying to decide
whether to kiss their forehead again
or leave before the traffic thickens,
you may not understand
that the leaving is its own kind of fracture.

If you have never driven home
after holding pressure on someone's life
and then held a toddler
who only wants an applesauce
and to mush your whole face—
you may not understand
how both requests
require everything.

They ask which matters more.
They ask how I choose.

If you have never held
two lives at once—
one in your arms,
one with your hands—
you may not understand
that the weight is the same,
but so is the love.
And love does not split.
It multiplies—
even when it costs sleep,
even when it costs certainty,

even when the world insists
you must be less of one
to be enough of the other.
I am not divided.
I am doubled.
And tomorrow
I will hold them both again.

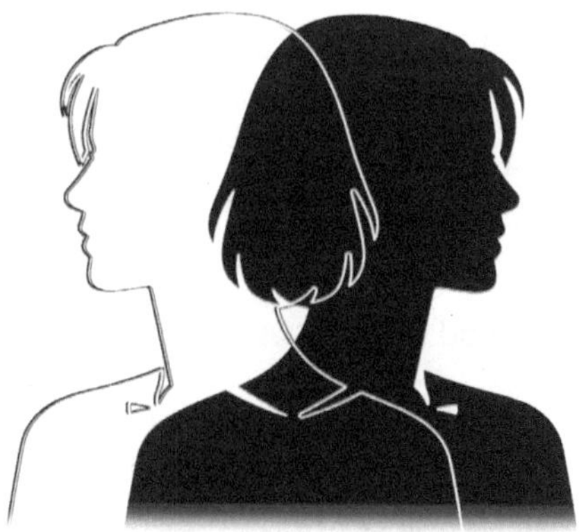

Metrics Can't Measure

Not burned out—
just burning through.
Not a flicker,
but a wildfire tearing through
red tape, silence, systems—
This is awakening.
You can't measure
what won't be contained:
heart, grit, defiance.
Yet we still show up,
for those trembling, looking
at us and seeing safety.
We know the fight
And still we rise.
Shift after shift,
charting after heartbreak—
we still rise.
Because they can't automate compassion.
They can't benchmark dignity.
They can't own the fire that keeps us human.
So lift your head.

Living Proof
that care still breathes,
that love still fights,
that no machine can do what you do
when you hold a hand like it matters.
We are burning brighter.

A Rainbow in Sight

A polite and practiced goodbye
waits with bated breath at the threshold,
uncertain of how it will be received.
The silence is the loudest confirmation
that it is time to soar—

The surrounding vines
have loosened their grip.
The ivory gate lay behind,
the horned gate ahead,
a rainbow in sight above,
trembles at the edge—
promise or memory,
it does not say.

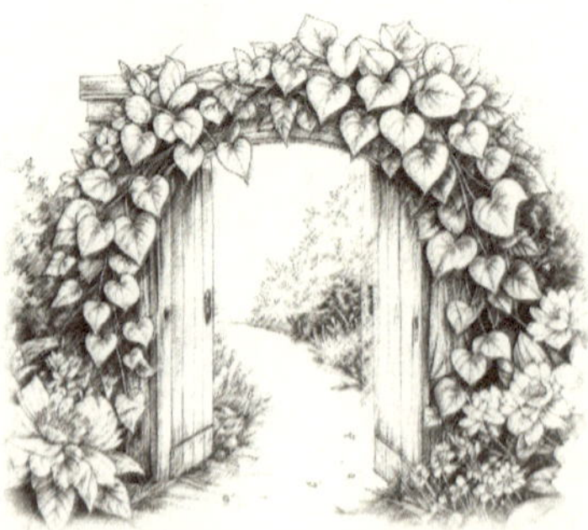

Movement

Sometimes fluid,
like thought learning to breathe.
Sometimes fractal,
truth repeating in smaller truths.
Sometimes linear,
a line drawn by memory.
Sometimes exponential,
becoming more than its beginning.
Sometimes spinning,
the self-seeking balance.
Sometimes twirling,
the soul remembering its dance.
Sometimes whirling,
between chaos and design.
Sometimes unfurling—
Always turning,
in motion and in mind,
each curve a quiet awakening.
Always turning,
and somehow,
the self moves deeper
into its own becoming

Squishmallow Heart

She gave a presentation, the teacher said,
about taking care of your heart.
Surprised, I asked her to tell me more.
At four years old she already knows
about transplants
about life and death.
She tells her friends,
eat more veggies,
move your bodies—
then you won't have to see my mom.
"She's a cardiomyopathy doctor," she says,
her chest puffed out with pride,
and from her backpack she pulls
a Squishmallow heart she'd hidden inside.
She could say cardiomyopathy
and LVAD by age two.
She even asks at night how
my patients are after I call.
She's learning empathy
from watching what I do.
I pray she keeps her wonder,
and her curious spirit, too.

In Good Standing

The wall gleams with framed affirmations.
Reputation hums through these corridors,
a quiet machinery of praise.
Care bends beneath the weight of billing.
A name becomes a number,
a story reduced to code.
Every doctor carries a graveyard
of patients in their head:
some tenderly,
some guiltily,
some unnamed—
their absence threaded through the silence.
We learned to chart the chemistry of pain,
to map cells, to trace the unseen—
but forgot the weight of a held gaze,
the quiet strength of simply being there.
Still, in the late hours,
kindness finds its secret corridors.
A hand steadies a hand,
a pause becomes its own medicine,
a glance holds what policies cannot.

Even here, amid the charts that never sleep,

the art survives—

fragile, defiant,

a small warmth insisting

it was never letters after a name,

but the courage to care beyond measure.

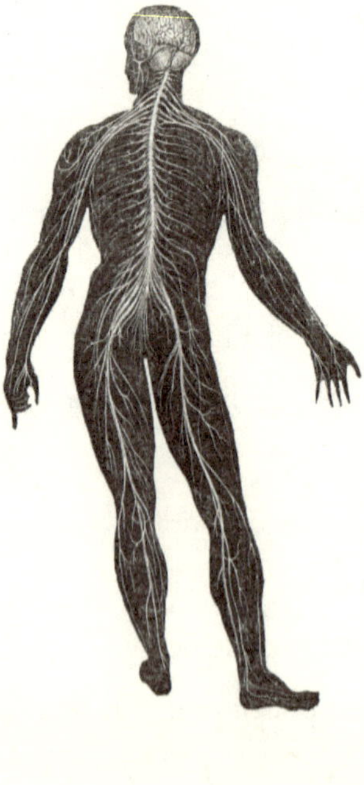

RVU

Three little letters.
They shouldn't matter,
but they live in the back of my mind,
whispering: not enough.
We were supposed to heal people.
That's what they told us.
But somehow it's become
a system that turns care into currency—
that sacred space between patient and doctor
reduced to lines on a billing sheet,
to numbers that claim to measure worth.
They call it productivity.
I call it survival.
Fifteen-minute visits.
Boxes to check.
Telling someone their heart is failing
while the next patient waits impatiently.
The patients keep getting sicker.
More tubes, more machines,
and somehow—minutes shrink.
I chase beeps and blinking screens
for 168 hours straight,

trying to remember
what it feels like to be human.
There used to be a golden age, right?
When care meant something more.
When we weren't so replaceable.
Sometimes I wonder if that world ever existed
or if it's just a story we tell ourselves
to keep from breaking.
Is it too much to want that back?
I think it might be.
Three little letters,
still whispering.

Ode to ______

Either a sorry or congratulations would be pretend—
The way it began could never predict its end.
A dance of wiggles, a quiet tug of war,
at times, no horizon visible from the shore.
Yet one thing stands unshaken and true:
the pattern of growth, threading all I've been through.
From this day forth, I claim my worth—
No longer bowed by moral distress or false rebirth,
I now climb steady toward new heights above the earth.

Scrubs at School

Wrinkled scrubs at dawn—
jam stains, pager's restless hum,
love beneath the rush

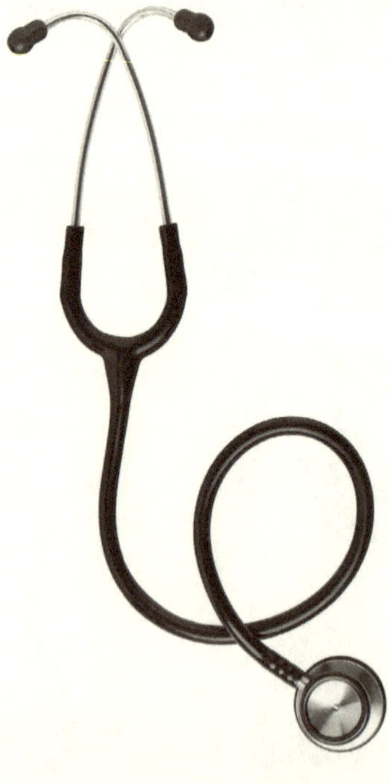

An ICU Elegy

The familiar beeps between the walls—
a cacophony turned reluctant symphony.
Someone needing,
something failing,
an organ whispering its last lament.

The familiar faces in this place—
a house of glass,
transparent yet concealed,
where every breath is both
confession and prayer.

The familiar scent that clings to air—
of flesh reborn and undone.
Lives rerouted in an instant,
checkmated by biology's hand.

The familiar touch in this exchange—
the pull of gravity,
the rise of hope,
the gentle armor of an encircling hug.

The familiar words—ritualistic and raw—
“Code blue.”
“I’m so sorry.”
“The time has come.”
Each phrase a closing door.

The familiar feelings in this sacred space—
grief, tension, joy, and grace intertwined.
Gratitude for all I’ve learned,
for all who’ve passed through my hands.
I carry you with me—
perhaps to return,
or to finally fly away.

Hope

So much hope—
It causes an awakening.
The air hums with promise,
grass dreams of green,
flowers ache to bloom,

the drought on the edge of
breaking.
Parched earth,
cracked and scorched,
screams with thirst,
begging for tomorrow,
when nothing is spared,
yet all may begin again.

Colliding forces—
whitewater to mist,
storm to silence—
rush then still.

The past carves its mark.
Mother Nature endures.
Beneath ice,
plates shift,
patient and unseen.
Change moves at the pace of stone.

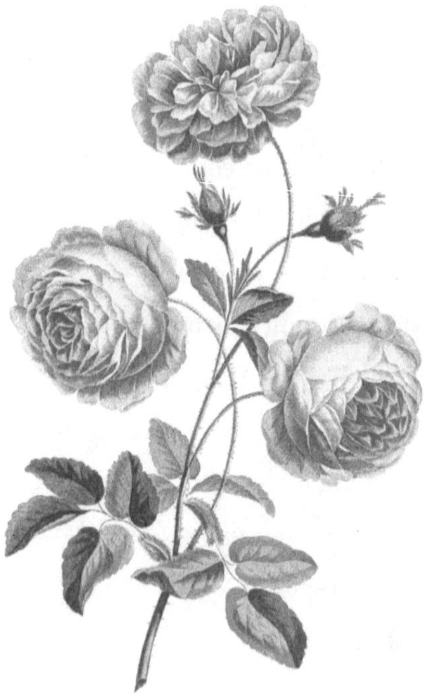

Resilient Cadence

Welcome aboard, you said—
"I'm proud of you. Keep it up."
Fresh eyes on a world our oyster.
No limit to what we can seize—
except when you fail to lead.
Spoken words vanish,
written ones erased,
and finding them again is like
squeezing water from stone.
Abandoned, stormy soul
is unharmed by being drowned.
Above ashes where roads once met,
the dove returns with empty claws—
in its place, a phoenix climbs.
Silence roars and truth thunders
beneath a blanket of stars.
There are no more echoes—
Hummingbird's resilient cadence sings.

Rhythm of Life

For years, a steady march—
Sinus rhythm.
Then suddenly, a screeching halt—

Ventricular fibrillation.
Start resuscitation.
Shock. Shock. Shock.
Epinephrine circulating.
Pulse check.
Barely alive,
hanging on by a thread—
ethereal, suspended.

The pendulum swings
between life and death,

A code blue lullaby.
Survival mode.
Sinus bradycardia.
Cardiac rehabilitation.
True realization.

"Stable," we say.
Live another day.
The scars might fade,
but never disappear.
Device check.
Goal-directed therapy.

Like a phoenix rising,
we rewrite the guidelines.

Ode to a Piece of Wood

This beautiful piece of wood that I play,
with curves so delicate and round and neat,
the notes that emanate from you each day,
are such a soulful and ethereal treat.

You sound best when showered with lots of love,
with much expression heard in your voice true,
Your feelings are as pure as two turtledoves,
every emotion can be shown through you.

You glorify humanity with grace,
strength that comes from both your soul and mind.
Although you seem as delicate as lace,
a tough trooper like you is hard to find.

Much can be done with a small little thing,
with a lovely violin with four beautiful strings.

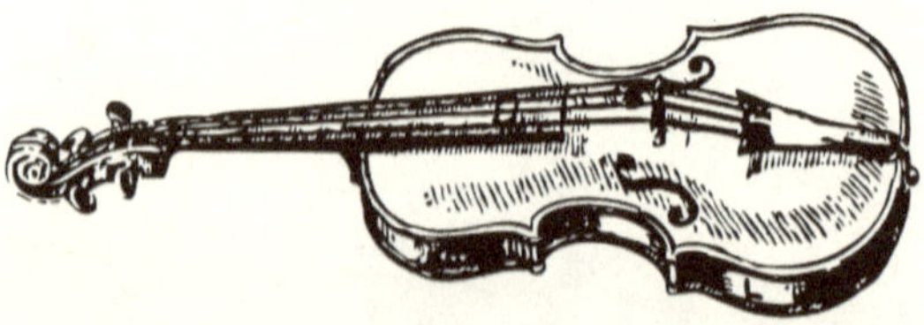

Superheroes

my little princess
in her Disney night gown
fighting a life-threatening illness
in her castle with a white tile floor
where the knights in shining armor
are the doctors in white coats

no white coat syndrome here
just people trying to save lives
even as a volunteer, I am already
her girlfriend, playing with Barbie
and pretty pony, sometimes a card game,
other times taking a trip
to "see the fishies" in the lobby

she basks in the little glories of life
in the hospital with pizza and Beetlejuice,
the last chemo banner decorates the door
i play my violin for her
and watch as her eyes sparkle
more than the world's most valuable jewel
a moment of pure elation for the two of us

SIX SIMPLE LETTERS

stab families
dripping with poison,
tearing them apart.

within thick tension
hearts crumble
under overwhelming fear
  is the end near?

no stone left unturned
sleepless nights of research
 hematology/oncology floor
 hospital clinic
 blood counts
 protocol
 treatment
 chemotherapy concoctions
 radiation
 —ironic, isn't it?
    saving lives with toxic poison

pray
share experiences
educate others
have faith
determination
optimism
laugh often
win the battle
make a wish
on a shining star
miracles= remission
  not so lucky
    relapse
precious time
   waiting stage
   nothing left unsaid
  pull closer together
sadness
   heart-wrenching
    deterioration
   why does this happen?

death
   same outcome either way
   a celebration of life

A LITANY FOR KIDS WITH CANCER

I am watching Princess Diaries two
pushing both a toy tractor and an iv pole
pulling a wagon, while
talking to someone my age
coloring pictures to give to nurses
playing Playstation 2
getting beaten at UNO several times
listening to a patient's story
finding out which life-threatening illness
a patient has been dealing with
giving parents a much-needed coffee break
rocking a premature baby
seeing the pain of a child with no hair
stuffing a dishwasher with filthy toys
hearing the sniffling of an exhausted family
loving a child whose parents never visit
unconditionally, living in the moment
saying "hi" to the security officers
connecting with a complete stranger
smiling with patients about their personal triumphs
cleaning a dirty playroom

helping a kid take their medicines
taking a patient to ultrasound
learning about the field of medicine
brightening the day of a tired doctor
with an enthusiastic "good morning"
assisting a nurse with a dressing change
believing in the power of faith and prayer
encouraging others to volunteer
making a difference
creating memories to last a lifetime
realizing that I am truly blessed
wishing that cancer didn't exist
thanking all the physicians, nurses, and volunteers
who helped me when I was in the hospital
thinking of myself as a future doctor
desiring to find a cure for cancer
playing my violin as "music therapy"
holding a two-year-old still for a finger stick
wondering how diseases came to be
finding myself amazed by modern medicine
turning on "Baby Mozart"
making the hospital a more cheerful place

Short White Coat

The once-gleaming short white coat is now
worn and multicolored. Spots of betadine,
hibiclens, and purell adorn each cuff.
Sleeves that now have permanent creases
from being rolled in just the same way
one too many times. The shoulder a tarnished
pink from the bag I carried each and every day.
Pockets stuffed to the brim with books, gloves,
IDs, and granola bars, the buttons have begun to fray,
the thread slowly unraveling

feeling at first so foreign,
now it feels comfortable,
a silent companion traveling with me,
sharing the firsts, the lasts, and the in-betweens,
helping bring new life into the world,
having discussions about terminal illness.
it became a sweatband, a tear-wiper,
a security blanket when entering the unfamiliar,
sometimes a real blanket when on call

Gently my fingers trace the emblazoned name
knowing that soon two more letters and a few more
inches will be added on like a butterfly
breaking free from the cocoon—a rebirth, of sorts
but also a death of this first coat
like an outgrown toy, fading
into a piece of nostalgia
while a new journey of growth begins again

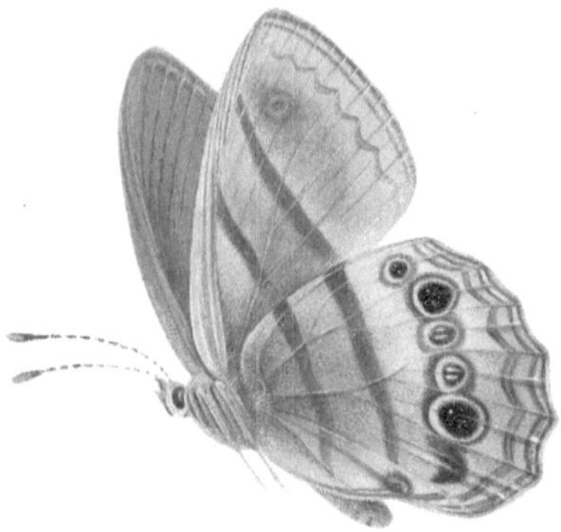

Borrowed Time

Tiny wisps of brown hair float freely
from her otherwise bald head,
a teddy bear tucked in her hand.
The scar across her head reminds us of the beast inside,
eating into the tissues viciously: a bloodthirsty monster
with no regard for anyone or anything.
It plays a tug of war with this girl's childhood,
back and forth: chemo, radiation, surgery.
Just watch and wait for it
to rear its ugly head again,
ripping away the childhood
to which she is entitled.
And yet through it all, she colors,
making artwork for the "sick kids,"
raising money for the pediatric cancer patients,
a group she doesn't include herself in.
She fills the world with love, with hugs, kisses,
and hope, dreaming of a cancer free world.

Cancer Hospital Expressway

It's morning rush hour
on the "cancer hospital expressway" elevators
a hustle and bustle pulsing with
people packed in like sardines—
white coats, raincoats, no coats
a symphony of pagers, cell phones, and iPods
many morning hellos and chatter
about the weather, our winning (or losing) teams,
the morning traffic. Steaming coffee in hand,
we scurry to see the patients
and race against the clock—
so much to do and so little time
ready to go back down we press
the silver button impatiently, the door
opens slowly, a fanfare of sorts—
there in front of my eyes a sobering reality:
the unmistakable metal cart
the white cloth pulled over
someone's final ride.
Such a dichotomy
the vibrancy of human interaction

the somber transport of a cadaver
at the same time in the same place
a little reminder to savor each moment
make holidays out of regular days
teach someone and pay it forward
all by 7:00 am at the hospital.

Silent Night

In the still of the night,
the soul sings so sweetly,
sharing its deepest desires through dreams.
The sky is a canvas dotted with twinkling stars—
We pray for serenity and guidance and the ability
To pair the dreams of the soul
With the reality of the world

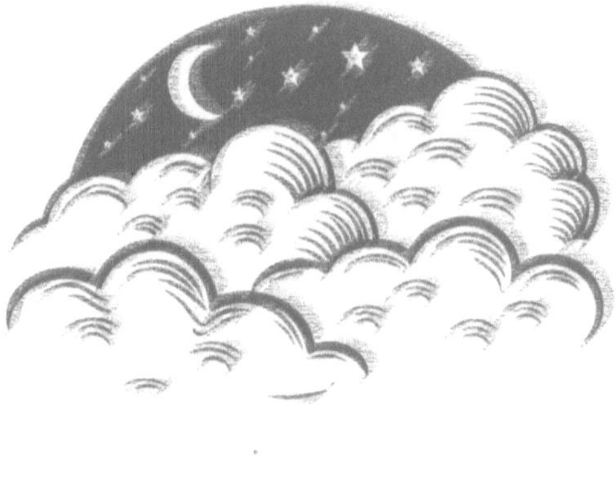

The cadaver speaks

I am a lifeless dreamer
You are my vitality
I am peaceful
You are my energy
I am a work of art
You are the museum curator
I am a fallen comrade
You are a soldier marching into battle
I am your textbook
You are the reader,
the one who must understand
I am your teacher
You are my student
I am your present (use me well)
You are the future

Hands

Your tiny hand is only big enough
to cover one of my fingers.
Your tight grasp amazes me—
How can one so little
have such a large impact on me already?
Your fingers ensnare mine
and our connection is forged,
a circle of trust
never to be broken.

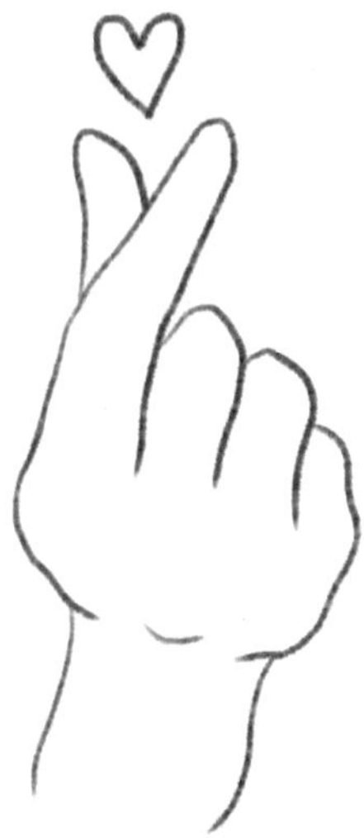

Midwestern Thanksgiving

Crackle crunch snap
The leaves rustle under my feet.
The trees are changing color—
Autumn is here.
The harvest is being picked,
apples and corn and pumpkins galore.
We shall gather together
with family and friends near and dear.
The birds are flying south,
The weather is getting cold,
Winter is near.

Family

A circle of trust,
close-knit and tight,
we are bound together by blood.
The learned and the learning,
the old and the young,
the teachers and the students,
the guru,
and the disciple—
all bridged together by time alone.

Little Angels

Curled up under soft fleece blankets
And warm quilts made with love
Children sleep quietly
Like angels
Dreaming of flying elephants and castles
And unicorns and roses
In a far off place
Where magic lives

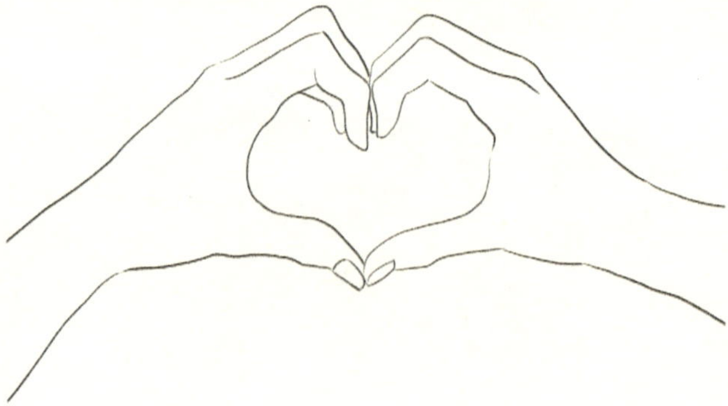

Circle of Life

The morning comes and the morning goes,
just as the night comes and the night goes.
So the days pass
swiftly yet slowly.
Time stops for no one—
Babies grow into adults,
the seasons change
from winter to spring
and summer to fall,
the sun rises and also it sets.
The years pass,
creating the circle of life

The Joys of Childhood

Putting sweaters on tomato plants
Eating huge chunks of cake too big to fit in your mouth
Pretending to play the violin with a notebook and a pencil
Carrying around a stuffed rabbit
Playing pretend with friends you love
Being the dog in a game of "house"
Sliding down a blue and yellow plastic slide
Jumping up and down on the trampoline
Playing hide and go seek in the dark
Getting piggyback rides and watching "Full House"
Moving Thomas the Tank Engine
Driving red hot wheels cars around
Going to the pool and belly flopping

Happiness

Hugs and kisses
Smiles and laughter
Being with family and friends
Baking ginger molasses cookies
Eating homemade food
Making chocolate almond mousse cake
Doing something nice for someone else
A smile on your face
Giving presents to others
Looking at old pictures of times past

Food of India

Makhani daal simmering in the slow cooker
Piping hot roti straight from the oven
Basmati rice bubbling on the stove
Spicy pickle that tickles your tongue
Gulab jamun that melts in your mouth
Papad so crisp that it breaks in your hand
Tamarind in the sambar that makes my lips pucker
Soft puffy idlis, little pillows of love
Savory and flavorful
Aromatic spices

I Love You

I love you stronger than the heaviest barbell.
I love you taller than the tallest skyscraper in the world.
I love you wiser than the smartest man on the planet.
I love you harder than the biggest granite block you can find.
I love you happier than the happiest person on earth.
I love you more than words can ever show.
I love you more than you will ever know.

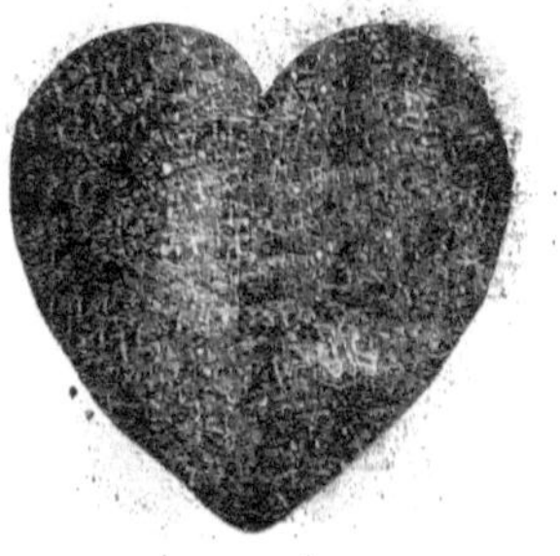

My Wish for You Is

Peace and joy,
Health and happiness,
The money to buy any toy.
My wish for you is
Good family and friends,
Comfort and Kindness,
A new path to follow when the first one dead-ends.
I wish for your love and trust,
Forgiveness and new beginnings,
And for all your life to be fair and just.
I wish for you strength and grace,
Courage and bravery,
And always a smile on your face.

Summer Rhythm

Fireflies dance in the warm air
Lighting up the nights
The day is long
The nights are short

Vacations and picnics
With watermelon and corn on the cob,
Barbecue and juicy meat rub,
And ice cold drinks wedged in a cooler.

Mosquito repellant and sunblock
Slathered behind hand-me-down sunglasses,
Skin baking to the color of warm wheat bread.

Relax and be carefree
Run barefoot through the grass
Bask in the rhythms of summer

Life, Unscripted

Garage doors
Kids
Crickets
Muddy shoes
Car horns
Doors
Traffic lights
Birds chirping
Rustling leaves
Streetlights
All settle down for a break.
Nighttime,
A moonlight serenade

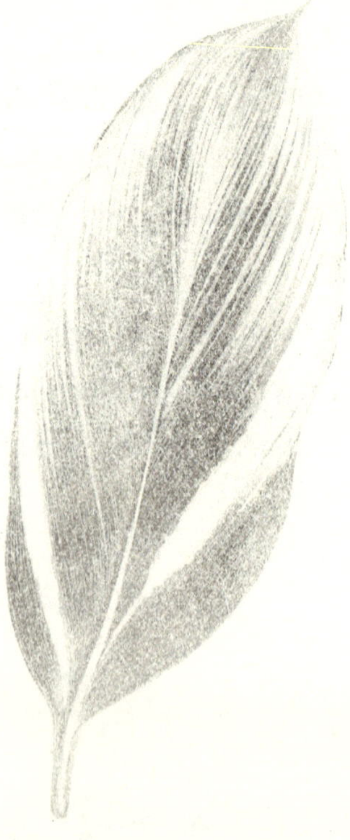

Snow Falling

Snowflakes dance in the starry night.
A dark sky becomes orange, purple, and white.
Each flake unique from all the others combines
into a dazzling beauty, creating a winter wonderland.
Yet massive strength and power make for raging storms.
Lightweight, airy, and fluffy, they are
like wisps of cotton balls pulled apart.
Simple yet so complex—
A natural phenomenon.

Time

Hold my hand and help me row—
Time will pass faster than you know.
Once I was young adorned with bows
Soon I'll be grown, showered in patients' woes.
The seasons change and the years pass.
Time stops for no one—
Not even the moon, the stars, or the sun.
So, enjoy each moment as if it were your last
because life comes at you all too fast.

Ocean

Calming waves of foam and water
Dig and sculpt the sand like a potter.
Gracefully and majestically
The power of nature is seen.
Water, vital to life itself,
So calm yet so furious
Raging and peaceful
Flowing freely and gently
Like a dress's apron billowing in the wind.
Sparkling and glinting in the sun
Crystal blue
Turquoise
Sea foam green
Pristine
Clear

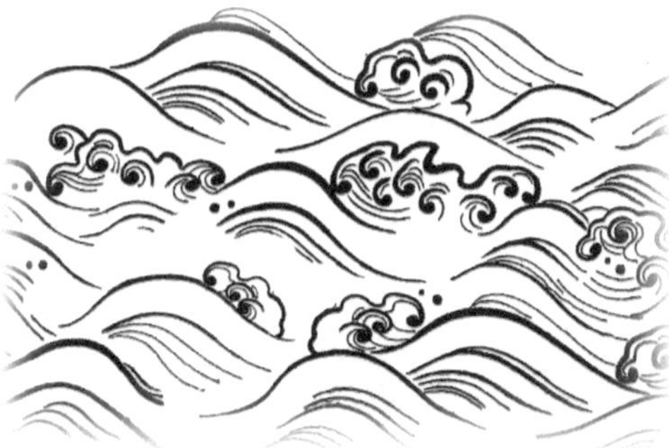

Connection

Do you ever wonder why I love you so much?
We are connected through blood and heart,
even though we are miles apart.
I think of you and your special touch—
I love you I love you I love you

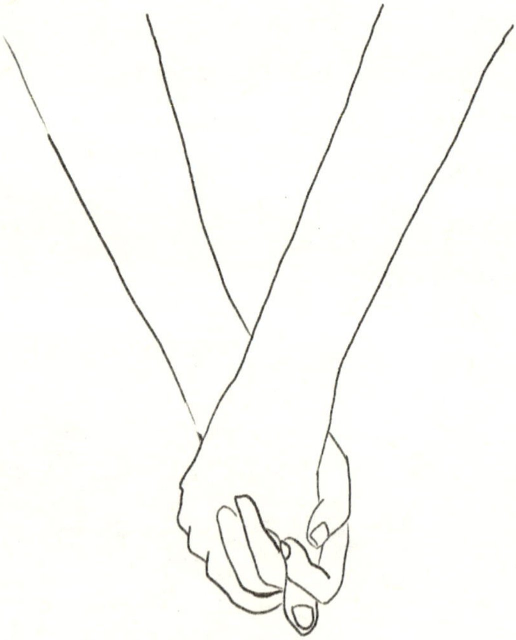

To My Parents

I can never show you the extent of my love
I am so blessed to call you my parents,
a gift from the universe above.
You are the most amazing role models in my life.
You have been by my side through success and strife.

My love can't be expressed with objects money can buy
So let me just say I'll love you till the day I die.
Instead of giving you a gift
with no meaning or one that will be forgotten fast,
I wrote you this poem, because I know it will last.
You mean the world to me and are always close to my heart.
In my life you have played such an instrumental part.
I love you so much—it grows each day.
I love you now and I will love you always

Orchestra

Like a swan on a crystal-clear lake
the parchment-colored horse hairs glide
across the sheep gut strings creating a sound
of angels in the heavens. Each push and pull
arouses such emotion, such beauty, such love
through elegant holes painstakingly carved into deep
mahogany wood. Melody lingers gently through the air
like the scent of a budding flower on a clean spring day.
How calming, how lovely, oh how the sounds are so sweet—
What a blessed and joyous treat.

How Much Do I Love You?

I love you more than all the twinkling stars at night.
I love you more than the buttery yellow sun shining so bright.
I love you more than cookies, candy, or cake.
I love you more than all the classes I diligently take.
I love you more than winter, spring, summer, and fall.
I love you more than the skyscrapers towering tall.
I love you more than the tallest tree.
I love you more than the loudest buzzing bee.
I love you more than the crystal blue lakes, rivers, and streams.
I love you more than chocolate raspberry truffle ice cream.
I love you more than all the April showers.
I love you more than any of the prettiest May flowers.
I love you more than I can show.
I love you more than you will ever know.

Bloom

Beautiful flower,
Open your bud
And grow.
Fill the world with color
And tickle my nose
with your delicate, sweet scent.

But you are fleeting, gone as quickly
and quietly as you came, like a ballet dancer,
flying through the air and landing offstage.

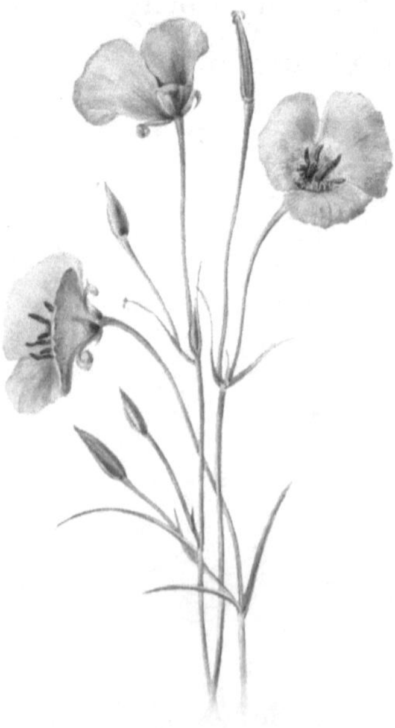

Angry

Heart pounding
Fist hammering
Temple throbbing
Vein bulging
Eye twitching
Face burning
Red Hot
Hot tamale

Calm

The wind rustling on a clear blue lake causes a ripple
No cars on the road
No screeching brakes
No traffic jam
No holiday rush
Leisurely strolls down the sidewalk
Birds chirping
Trees swaying gently in the breeze

Niagara

Whitewater rapids,
Thundering and massive
Booming
Falls of frigid water.
Natural power of nature,
Making energy,
Creating rainbows in the mist.
Get as close as you can to feel the rain
on your skin. Feel the push and pull of nature.
Get swept by the gusts of wind
Experience the beauty and the magnificence

Special Moments

Warm feelings in your heart and all around,
Knowing that you brightened someone's day
Realizing the goodness of yourself and others.
Understanding that someone cares
To dance to the music you helped create.
Smiling at others no matter how different they seem,
Singing and creating memories together,
Remembering those times even when loved ones are gone,
Changing feelings, attitudes, and outlooks,
Sharing a smile, encouragement, little as it may be,
Crying to comfort wounds so deep,
Laughing at one another's vices and follies,
Taking time to connect,
And creating special bonds that last a lifetime.

Blessed to Call You My Own

Brush my hair
Hold me tight
Sing me a song
Tuck me in goodnight
Take away the monsters from under my bed
Make my favorite food for me
Kiss away the boo-boo that is on my head
Come sit and sip some pretend tea
Go on an adventure with me to a faraway land
Don't let me go, please hold my hand
Be my playmate, caretaker, and best friend all in one
I love you mom
And you love me
You do more for me than anyone can see
I love you more than anything in the world
You are more valuable than any gemstone.
I'm so blessed to call you my own.

You Will Always Be in My Heart

I walked into the unknown
ready to prove to others why
I wanted to be "the one."
And there you were,
sitting on the black leather couch,
awaiting your chance as well.
It was as though I knew you
before I met you. Rather, I knew
I would like you, and yet it was joyful.

The unexpected pleasure of a newborn friendship,
one that would grow and grow for years to come,
unbeknownst to either of us at that time.
Together our journeys interwove for a period of time.
You and I made footprints and cast shadows
in the Ohio sunshine, heat, rain, and snow.

Now as our roads diverge once more
I know we'll continue to share our special connection.
It will be preserved like the grand prize-
winning canned peaches of the state fairs,
Like an antique heirloom passed down through the generations.
I know we'll be there for each other until the end.

Reflections on Geriatrics

She was fragile and frail,
sitting in a bed three times her size,
speaking in a language known only to herself.
There was no recognition of who
we were or why we were there. To her
my white coat and stethoscope were meaningless.
Though she could not see,
she reached out to grasp my hand,
gingerly stroking each finger,
gently feeling the ridges of my knuckles,
as if taking a picture of me in her mind.
Our hands intertwined, and in that moment,
through a connection without spoken words,
I saw the beauty of geriatric medicine

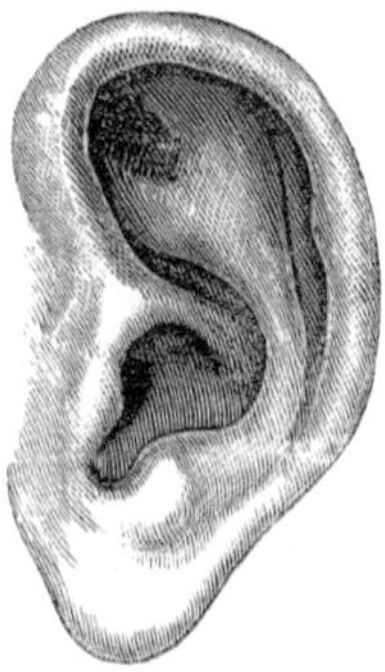

The Reason for Going Into Medicine

"I just finished my first year of med school" I said.
The resident instructed, "Say you are starting the second instead."

"What do you see here?" the pathologist asks
I think of squiggly lines and ulcers shaped like a flask.

"Describe this film" the radiologist points
As I try to decipher each bone and each joint.

"What are the drug interactions" the pharmacist questions
Oh my I'm feeling the tension!

The surgeon tells me to adjust the light
I do it quickly and quietly to avoid any fights.
I try my best, with all my might.

Time goes by, day by day,
Those days and nights they fly away.
I've gone through all my rotations now,
Now I've got to pick just one.... But how?
There are things that I've loved about every single one,

But certainly a few that I'm glad to have done.
I want to choose something I'll love for years to come,
Something that will make my life full of fun.

"Go see the patient on your own" the attending said,
"Are you sure about this?" was going through my head.

I tentatively knock with my clammy hand,
smoothing my oversized coat, feeling like a contraband.

Nervously I step forward as the "come in" is heard.
Excited to finally get to "be a real doctor," I find my nerve.

"Be confident be confident be confident" I think.
I hope this patient doesn't tell the others I stink.

Calmly I go through the steps I've rehearsed in the past,
trying to be steady, not too slow or too fast.

She tells me the problems she's been having with her knee,
the struggles she has had following the latest surgery.

Upset and frustrated with her body and its lack of motion,
she begins to cry and freely shares her emotions.

"Whoa," I thought, I was not expecting this first test.
I guess I will have to try my best.

The Kleenex were found and I rolled my chair near.
I held her hand and just listened with both ears.

"You are a good doctor," she says,
"Thank you for being there for me."
"Oh you know I'm just a student…" I stammer.
She'll never know that she was the first,
the first patient I saw by myself,
the first patient that cried to me,
the first patient to thank me for helping her.

But I'll keep her tears and her story in my heart
to remember that I can make a difference,
to remember to listen,
to remember to be the best I can be,
to remind myself why I went into medicine.

Night Shift

Evening has fallen,
visiting hours are over.
We sit in our scrubs,
pockets stuffed with notes and snacks.
The night is still young.
Pagers continuously croon.
The list of tasks grows.
Our bodies grow weary.

Oh, what we would do
to be able to shut our eyes
for a glorious minute or two.

Suddenly, we hear it,
like the shot heard 'round the world.
The pager now blares
Code Blue! Code Blue!
We hear it overhead too.
Like cheetahs, we race to the room
and spring into action.

There is no chaos of a TV medical drama
or your normal Friday Night Lights.
There is no time to drive down the field—
We must punt now and pray,
tear off the white coat and throw on the gloves.
I'm only a medical student,
but now, I'm an able body with willing hands.
I clasp my hands together and lock my elbows
to compress the chest. They taught us to think about
the BeeGees to keep the pace. How ironic to think about
Staying Alive as we try to keep a mother,
daughter, sister, aunt, and grandmother from dying.

Eclipse

Clouds veil
The lunar eye.
I wake
Beneath the arc of totality,
Hoping against hope
To see,
To connect
With the cosmos
Near the lion's fading roar of stars.
But alas, too many clouds,
Too much light—
The dragons prevail.

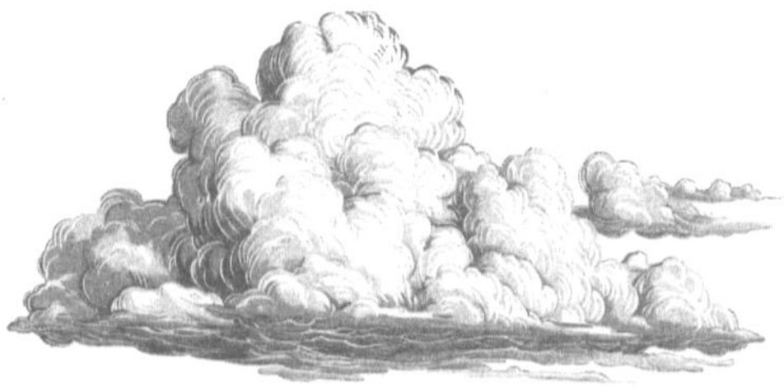

Morning has broken

A spring awakening
Refreshed, renewed —
Growth unfurls in golden hush.
How magical it is for light to linger,
Squeezing into every nook and cranny,
Drops of daylight spill and sway,
Painting warmth on waking skin.
In every glimmer — a promise waking,
The world beginning again in light.

Housewarming

Something borrowed,
Something true.
A place of change,
A place of love,
A place of hope,
A place we've been dreaming of.
Time to come,
Time to go,
Time to flow,
Time to grow.
A second to spare,
A minute to wait,
A day at a time,
A year flies by.
Yet here we stand,
Both tried and new,
Love our compass,
Guiding through.
May this home be filled with light,
Morning joy and stars at night.
Walls that echo love's embrace,

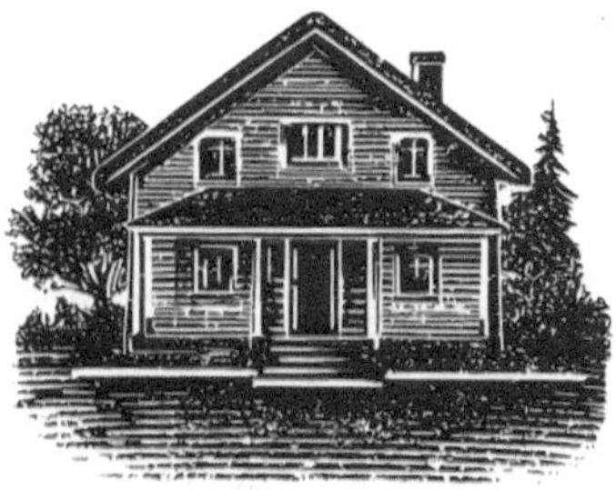

Windows shining grace on grace.
May laughter dwell in every room,
And kindness chase away all gloom.
May friends feel welcome at the door,
And leave with hearts a little more.
Let patience root and hope be grown,
Peace reside in every stone.
Through every season, come what may,
Love will guide and light the way.

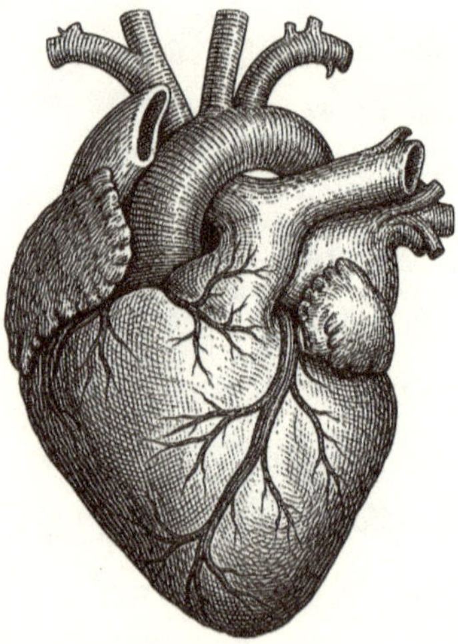

The Time Has Come

The time has come
to step into a new chapter—
one that's waited for you
with arms wide as dawn.
The time has come
to leave this place
that kept your laughter,
your quiet, your ache.
The time has come
to walk unmarked paths,
a compass steady in your chest—
you've always known the way.
The time has come
to close this door softly,
the universe whispering
its prayer of peace.
The time has come
to burn ahead, alive,
chasing joy like fire
through the open fields.
The time has come
to stand still
with a grateful heart,
and listen for the light

Home

Home is a concept.
Home is a feeling.
Home is being with your loved ones.
Home is for framily and friendsgiving.
Home is making things your own,
wherever you find yourself.
Home is exploring—
discovering comfort in new corners.
Home is shokupan in the oven,
a hot masala dosa,
chocolate chip cookies from Mom's recipe.
Home is unconditional love that doesn't ask.
Home is patience that waits.
Home is support that never fades.
Home is not a place—
it's the love you live in,
it's the comfort you carry
wherever you go.

A Sky Full of Stars

You are never alone—
a guardian angel flies by your side.
Once there were two,
but you became the chosen one.
The reason still hides in the vast unknown,
a question the stars cannot explain.
Still, I believe this much is true:
you are thriving now,
held by that unseen protection.

A Breath of Fresh Air

A hummingbird takes flight,
Sipping sweet nectar
Before the next journey.
Wings whisper quickly,
Effortless in the air.
A piece of coal,
With time
And a little space,
Turns into something
That holds the light.
A gradual crescendo,
The orchestra rising,
Grows to brightness—
The air itself becomes song,
Weightless, lifting everything.

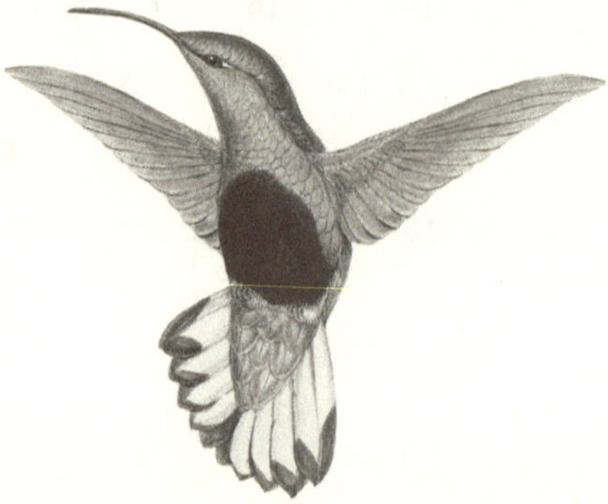

To Listen

Listen, child, and do not speak.
You will learn so much more
When you pause,
Take a breath,
And feel the stillness settle around you.
Look, and notice the difference
Between what is seen and what is heard —
The intricate metaphors,
The delicate similes,
The tone that carries meaning softly through the dark.
Be patient with the world's small sounds,
The pace of every voice,
And in your quiet observations,
Let understanding bloom.

Holding Space

I sit beside your storm,
neither steering nor stilling it—
only breathing with the tide,
waiting for the calm to find its own shore.
Words would ripple the water,
so I choose silence instead,
an open field where your truth
can unfurl without pruning.
I meet you where you are—
not at the edge of fixing,
but at the heart of being,
where every wound is already learning light.
In this slowing,
you soften into yourself,
begin to see the wholeness hiding
in the kernels you once called broken.
All that you seek
has been waiting, quietly,
in the space you've made
by finally letting yourself be.

The autopsy

Dead and festered—
Yet you couldn't bear to be alone,
Hiding beneath invisible armor,
Your mask too thin to hide the ruin.
Hollow, empty,
You didn't even listen.
Had you heard,
You might have felt
My palpitations—
A thready pulse,
A rhythm you never noticed.
Apathetic, emotionless—
I knew better,
And still, I believed
That maybe you would see me.
But stone,
You remained.
The dust settles.
Postmortem complete.
Cause of death: natural.
And so I whisper my own benediction—
May I be happy.
May I be healthy.
May I be at peace.
May I be at ease.

Anniversary

One year has passed.
Should I blow out the candles,
Say congratulations—
Or grieve for what has changed,
Not for what was lost,
For not everything gone was worth keeping.
Do I trace the scars,
Feel the sinewy stretch of healing skin,
Or keep the bandage on,
Because the ache still throbs beneath?
I have walked through fire,
Stepped barefoot on coals,
And now each turn around the sun
Feels heavier—
And somehow lighter too.
A slow, choreographed dance
Toward the faint shimmer of possibility.
Step out, beautiful one,
From the oven's inferno.
You are the ocean's breath now—
Calm, cool,

A rainbow risen from the mist,
Pressure released,
Time your own again.
So yes—
Perhaps I can celebrate this
As a rebirthing day,
Singing a different tune,
Whispering gratitude to the universe
For this perfectly imperfect wholeness,
This raw brilliance—
A complete gem,
Still shining.

I Am The Hero of My Journey

I am the hero of my journey
Someone who has woven a rich tapestry of experiences,
creating meaning,
reflecting,
pausing.
I am the hero of my journey—
daring myself to achieve greater heights,
finding a path when nothing is visible,
creating light from darkness,
choosing myself.
I am the hero of my journey,
strong-willed and powerful,
the fledgling sapling that persisted,
unafraid to try,
desperate to grow.
I am the hero of my journey—
becoming, unfolding,
still writing the story,
still reaching toward the sun.
I am the hero of my journey.

Manifest Destiny

Not in the number of papers I write,
But in the stories I've truly lived.
Not in the letters behind my name,
But in the moments I gave my time.
Not in the balance of my bank account,
But in the fullness of my spirit.
Not in the titles I've held,
But in the care I've offered to myself and others.
To live deeply.
To love deeply.
To experience fully.
This is how I wish to live.

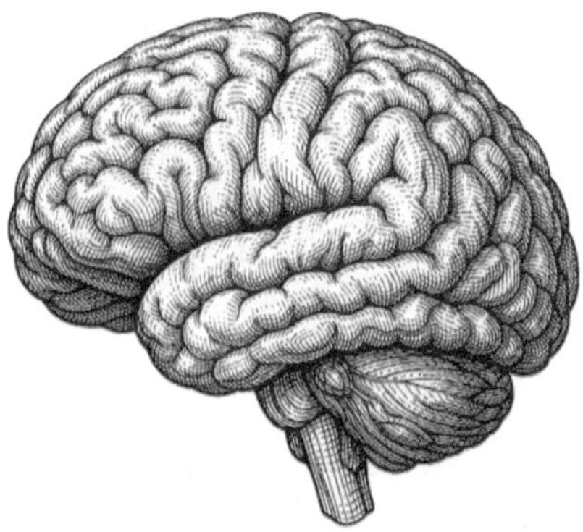

Tale of Two Pumps

In the LVAD storage room, hums intertwine—
one tugging milk, one pushing blood through steel.
Both pulse in rhythm with what it means to live,
to nurture, to mend, to keep the fragile whole.
The click and whir of duty never pause,
whether for patient, child, or self.
Hands learning new rhythms, from pulse to pump,
guiding the flow, turning motion into nourishment.
The circle turns—
Life sustained by circuitry and love.
Machines mimic hearts; a mother becomes one,
feeding both science and infancy, unseen.
Exhaustion seeps through scrubs and skin,
but in this hidden corner, there's grace.
Two pumps, steady and sure,
reminding what all this work is for—
a heartbeat here, a heartbeat there—
and the rhythm of creation unbroken.

Author's Note: This was written by the author as a reflection on her journey in medicine, 3 decades after the initial 3rd grade writing

I Am

I am the woman who learned how heavy healing can be.
I wonder how that brave, wide-eyed girl would see me now.
I hear the cries that echo through crowded waiting rooms.
I see those who arrive late because buses run slow and life runs hard.
I want to ease their suffering, even when I cannot cure it.
I am the woman who learned how heavy healing can be.
I feel the weight no textbook ever warned me about.
I touch hands that tremble between life and loss.
I worry my voice is too small against a system built on silence.
I cry—quietly now—for the ones I cannot save or even reach.
I am the woman who learned how heavy healing can be.
I understand that some pain has no cure and some wounds are written in history.
I try to make people feel seen in a world that often looks away.
I hope my presence offers dignity where power runs thin.
I know the little girl became the doctor she promised she would be—and she has learned that healing is more than curing.
I am the woman who learned how heavy healing can be.

www.ingramcontent.com/pod-product-compliance
Lightning Source LLC
LaVergne TN
LVHW100324210926
848480LV00003B/1251
* 9 7 9 8 9 9 6 1 6 0 2 1 1 *